Unlike other valuable antioxidants, lipoic acid is both water- and fat-soluble, so can be used throughout the body. It enhances the effect of other antioxidants and helps them resist being used up as they defend the body against free-radical damage. This concise but comprehensive guide shows how lipoic acid is effective against diabetes, heart disease and toxic metals, and even shows action against the HIV virus that causes AIDS.

LIPOIC ACID: THE METABOLIC ANTIOXIDANT

ISBN: 0-87983-720-9

Printed in the United States of America

Keats Good Health Guides™ are published by
Keats Publishing, Inc.
27 Pine Street (Box 876)
New Canaan, Connecticut 06840-0876

Contents

ABOUT THE AUTHOR

Richard A. Passwater, Ph.D. is one of the most called-upon authorities in preventive health care. A noted biochemist, he is credited with popularizing the term "supernutrition" in such books as *Supernutrition: Megavitamin Revolution* and *The New Supernutrition.* His many other works include *Cancer Prevention and Nutritional Therapies* and *Pycnogenol.* Dr. Passwater lives in Berlin, Maryland, where he is the director of a research laboratory.

Lipoic Acid: The Metabolic Antioxidant

The unique nutrient that recharges energy levels and the body's defenses

Richard A. Passwater, Ph.D.
Author of Supernutrition for Healthy Hearts

Keats Publishing, Inc. New Canaan, Connecticut

WHY ALL THE EXCITEMENT?

Nutritional scientists are very excited today about a once obscure nutrient, lipoic acid. What is lipoic acid and why all the excitement? Lipoic acid is a key compound for producing energy in muscles and an important link in the vital antioxidant network. It is an essential "key" that unlocks the energy from food calories. Lipoic acid directs calories into energy production and away from fat production. The energy produced is available not only for moving the skeletal muscles, but for everything we need to do. When we improve our efficiency to produce energy, we improve our ability to perform at top level in everything we do from exercising to thinking.

Lipoic acid normalizes blood sugar levels and reduces glycation, the damage sugar does to critical body components. This damage leads to accelerated aging, heart disease and the adverse effects of diabetes.

Although there are hundreds of studies over forty years revealing how lipoic acid energizes metabolism, the new excitement about this nutrient can be seen in the many recent studies focusing on how it improves the physique, combats free radicals, protects our genetic material, slows aging, helps protect against heart disease, cancer and many other diseases.

Both insulin-dependent and non-insulin dependent diabetics will be excited to learn that lipoic acid has been used for nearly thirty years in Europe to treat diabetic neuropathy, help regulate blood sugar, and prevent diabetic retinopathy and cardiopathy. Lipoic acid not only protects the nervous system, but may be involved in regenerating nerves as well. It is also being studied in the treatment of Parkinson's disease and Alzheimer's disease.

Lipoic acid has also been used for decades to protect the liver and to detoxify the body of heavy metal pollutants. One of the most exciting recent developments is that lipoic acid appears to help slow the progression of HIV infection to clinical AIDS. This is not important only to HIV-positive people, but to all of us, as AIDS treatment adds billions of dollars to our health costs which we all pay either as increased insurance premiums or taxes.

We make some lipoic acid in our bodies, but usually not enough, so we depend on food to get what we need for optimal health. This means that it is not quite a vitamin by definition, but is classified as the very next thing to a vitamin. Lipoic acid is also a "conditionally essential" antioxidant nutrient. Conditionally essential simply means that it is essential to life, but that young healthy people normally don't have to get all of it from food. Since our ability to make lipoic acid in our bodies tends to decline with age or disease, many people don't produce enough and their health becomes very dependent on how much they get in their diet.

Lipoic acid's antioxidant function is of major imortance. Antioxidant nutrients help protect the body against the damage that can cause heart disease, cancer, aging and about eighty other diseases. This damage is caused by undesirable by-products of metabolism called free radicals. Not only does lipoic acid improve metabolism, it protects us against the harmful by-products of metabolism.

Lipoic acid both interacts with its antioxidant partners, vitamin E and vitamin C, and helps conserve them. When the body is deficient in lipoic acid, the other antioxidants do not properly network together.

Lipoic acid also protects the liver and detoxifies tissues of heavy metals such as excessive iron and copper, and the toxic metals cadmium, lead, and mercury.

It is amazing that a single nutrient has so many actions. The value of lipoic acid to our health is best described by its nickname: the metabolic antioxidant. Lipoic acid is a coenzyme that is involved in metabolism (energy production) and a universal antioxidant that directly and indirectly helps protect every body component from the damage of oxidative stress.

SUGGESTED READING

1. Alpha-lipoic acid as a biological antioxidant. Packer, L., Witt, E. H., and Tritschler, H. J. Free radical Biol. & Med. 19(2):227–50 (1995)
2. Lipoic acid basics. Passwater, Richard A. Whole Foods (January 1996)

A DUAL HISTORY—METABOLISM AND ANTIOXIDANT

As long ago as 1951 lipoic acid attracted the interest of scientists who specialized in elucidating the roles of B-complex vitamins, because of its action as an essential coenzyme. A coenzyme is a nonprotein substance that combines with a protein to form a complete enzyme. An enzyme is a protein that speeds up reactions or makes it possible for certain reactions to occur in the body. Enzymes are not consumed in the reactions that they facilitate. Most human coenzymes are produced from some of the B-complex vitamins or are themselves vitamins.

At one time, lipoic acid seemed to be a member of the vitamin B complex. Lipoic acid seemed to be destined to become the first fat-soluble vitamin B isolated. But, as I noted earlier, lipoic acid is not a "true" vitamin because the body can make enough to prevent a recognizable deficiency disease (though not enough to perform all its functions, hence its "conditionally essential" status). As a coenzyme, lipoic acid has an advantage over most true vitamins, which have to be converted into coenzymes.

Early clues to the function of lipoic acid suggested that it was a catalyst with high biological activity required for the oxidation of carbohydrates and fatty acids which leads to the generation of ATP. A catalyst is an element or compound that facilitates a reaction that might not otherwise occur to a significant extent without its help. Enzymes are catalysts that the body needs to carry out the thousands of biochemical reactions in the body needed for controlling the life process.

The generation of ATP is critical. ATP (adenosine triphosphate) is the compound that stores energy in the body. Energy is a force, not a compound, but energy can be stored in various ways, physically and chemically. The body stores energy in ATP and then releases when it's needed.

Lipoic Acid the Antioxidant

It was realized fairly early that lipoic acid also served as a biological antioxidant when researchers found that it prevented scurvy in vitamin C deficient animals, and by 1988 it began to emerge as a universal antioxidant with many properties.

After the original flurry of research on lipoic acid as a coenzyme, interest faded when it looked doubtful that it was dietarily essential. Eventually it was noted that lipoic acid entered into a relationship with glutathione that protected cell components against lipid peroxidation. This was discovered by Drs. A. Bast and G. Haenen in 1988.

Dr. Lester Packer of the University of California at Berkeley is a pioneer in the research on lipoic acid as an antioxidant. In 1991, he found it to be an important part of a network of antioxidants that includes vitamin C, vitamin E and glutathione. In 1993, Dr. Packer found that lipoic acid also functions to protect a key nuclear factor that is involved in the expression and regulation of genes. This has major implications for our health and will be discussed in detail later.

Summary

Thus, as the metabolic antioxidant, lipoic acid is multifunctional. It is essential for energy production, and provided enough is available in the body, it can act as a powerful antioxidant.

Suggested Reading

1. Snell, E. E., Tatum, E. L. and Peterson, W. H. J. Bact. 33:207 (1937)

2. Guirard, B. M., Snell, E. E. and Williams, R. J. Arch. Biochem. 9:381 (1946)

3. Crystalline alpha-lipoic acid: A catalytic agent associated with pyruvate dehydrogenase. Reed, L. J, DeBusk, B. G., Gunsalus, I. C. and Hornberger, Jr., C. S. Science 114(2952):93–4 (1951)

4. Multienzyme complexes. Reed, L. J. Accounts Chem. Res. 7:40–46 (1974)

5. Interplay between dihydrolipoic acid and glutathione in the protection against microsome lipid peroxidation. Bast, A. and Haenen, G. Biochem. Biophys. Acta 963:558–61 (1988)

6. Antioxidant action of thioctic acid and dihydrolipoic acid. Kagan, V., Khan, S., Swanson, C., Shevedova, A., Serbinova, E. and Packer, L.

   Free Rad. Biol. Med. 9S:15 (1990)

7. Reactive oxygen intermediates as apparently widely used messengers in the activation of NF-kappa-alpha. Shreck, R., et al. EMBO J. 10:2247–58 (1991)

THE "ESSENTIAL" BASICS

The chemical structure of lipoic acid gives it unique capabilities. It consists of a relatively small, eight-member chain having two sulfur atoms, one attached to the sixth carbon atom and the other sulfur atom attached to the eighth carbon atom, with the sulfurs also linked to each other which results in a ring. The molecular weight of lipoic acid is 206. The high-energy sulfur atoms are largely responsible for lipoic acid's ability to function in three important ways:

1) as a coenzyme in the energy process,
2) as a powerful antioxidant, and
3) as a chelator to remove excess iron and copper, and toxic metals such as cadmium, lead and mercury.

We know how unique the structure of the compound is, but we don't know very much about how this complex compound is assembled in the body, so we don't know what the limiting factors are for its biosynthesis. When I asked Dr. Jim Clark of the Henkel Corporation, he suggested that it is synthesized from an eight carbon carboxylic acid called octanoic acid. Dr. Clark also suggested that the sulfur atoms come from cysteine, a sulfur-containing amino acid, but the exact chemical mechanism and the factors that control the synthesis are not known yet. This suggests to me that a dietary deficiency of sulfur-containing amino acids would limit the production of lipoic acid, but there are other nutritional factors and diseases that also interfere with lipoic acid production.

As I mentioned earlier the body does not make enough lipoic acid for optimal health. The optimal level of lipoic acid varies from person to person depending on biochemical individuality, lifestyle, and especially how much exercise and oxidative stress they experience. Age, disease and environmental conditions that increase oxidative stress can cause a deficiency in lipoic acid, so that the body can't make enough to meet all its metabolic and antioxidant needs. There is a lot of evidence that the body makes barely enough for its metabolic needs and does not produce enough for optimal antioxidant needs. The additional lipoic acid needed for antioxidant functions must come from dietary sources, including supplements. In some stressful situations it is necessary to get lipoic acid for both optimal metabolic function and antioxidant functions via the diet. This, again, is why lipoic acid is considered "conditionally essential."

Both Water- and Fat-Soluble

One of the reasons that lipoic acid is so versatile is that it can go virtually anywhere in the body to function. It is a rare nutrient in that it is compatible with—and soluble in—both water-based and fat-based components of the body. There are only two systems of solubility—polar and nonpolar. This translates into plain English as water-soluble and fat-soluble.

Lipoic acid's dual solubility is a main reason that it is sometimes referred to as a universal antioxidant, as well as the metabolic antioxidant. It is not as water-soluble as vitamin C, but it is much more water-soluble than vitamin E. Its degree of water-solubility and fat-solubility allows lipoic acid entry into all body systems. The main reason for this dual solubility is the size of the molecule. With a molecular weight of 206, it is larger than ascorbic acid (molecular weight of 176) but much smaller than vitamin E (molecular weight of 431).

A second factor is the functionality of the molecule. It does contain a carboxylic acid end-group, and that has a tendency to make it more soluble in water than vitamin E. At the same time it has more carbon atoms than vitamin C and that makes it more soluble in lipid compartments.

THE SULFUR ATOMS ARE THE KEY

The chemical structure of lipoic acid is a simple molecule having a "backbone" of eight carbon atoms. Nature, instead of adding a hydroxyl group to form a monophenol nutrient like vitamin E, or adding several hydroxyl groups similar to bioflavonoids, adds two sulfur atoms and links them together. Sulfur atoms have a lot to do with lipoic acid's function as a coenzyme.

Lipoic acid is a cofactor in what is called a multienzyme complex. The lipoic acid itself is bound to a very complex enzyme which is a high-molecular weight protein. As such, it is not consumed when it is serving as a metabolic cofactor but is continually regenerated.

The process gets rather complex. But when lipoic acid is in its role of a metabolic coenzyme, the carboxylic acid end-group anchors it to the enzyme through formation of a chemical bond called an "amide linkage" or a "peptide linkage."

The sulfur atoms are critical to the action of lipoic acid as an enzyme, and also keys to lipoic acid being a powerful and versatile antioxidant.

SULFUR MAKES LIPOIC ACID A POWERFUL ANTIOXIDANT

Adding to the versatility conveyed by lipoic acid's dual solubility is the fact that it also cycles between its oxidized and reduced forms, which are both powerful biological antioxidants. The fact that lipoic acid has a ring structure having a sulfur-sulfur linkage that can split, breaking the ring, and allow hydrogen to be added to the sulfur atoms has much to do with the antioxidant function of the molecule. The oxidation potential between the sulfur-sulfur bond and the sulfur-hydrogen bond is such as to allow easy interconversion under physiological conditions. The tissues can quite easily convert lipoic acid, which has a sulfur-sulfur bond, to dihydrolipoic acid, which has cleaved that sulfur-sulfur bond and replaced it with two sulfur-hydrogen bonds.

In allowing this hydrogen addition to the sulfur atoms, lipoic acid can cycle back and forth between the two forms—lipoic acid and dihydrolipoic acid. This is called "redox cycling." Redox cycling is simply the interconversion of an oxidized form of the material to a reduced form and back again. In some materials, the oxidation or reduction is irreversible. But the reduction and oxidation of lipoic acid is quite reversible; it can sit there and switch from one to the other. This is a real advantage because it allows it to act as a carrier, as a transfer agent for electrons from one compound to another.

The two forms have different chemical functionalities and can react in different ways with other materials. Compounds that supply hydrogen atoms or electrons in chemical reactions are called reducing agents. Oxidizing agents are compounds that receive hydrogen atoms or electrons. The primary difference is the fact that the reduced form—the dihydrolipoic acid—is a much stronger reducing agent and it is capable of regenerating vitamin C and vitamin E from their oxidized forms.

SULFUR HELPS REMOVE TOXIC METALS

It is apparent that lipoic acid is itself a versatile and direct antioxidant. However, there is still more to its antioxidant protective actions. It also has an indirect action via its ability to remove toxic metals and excessive minerals.

SUMMARY

1. Lipoic acid has a unique structure that gives it many special actions.
2. Lipoic acid is both water-soluble and fat-soluble.
3. Its sulfur atoms are the key to its coenzyme function, antioxidant function and chelating function.
4. Lipoic acid is not technically a vitamin, but it is so important to the body that the body makes some. However, lipoic acid is "conditionally essential," meaning that most people may not make enough in their bodies for optimal health.
5. Lipoic acid is well absorbed and transported into the cells where it does its many jobs.

THE METABOLIC ENERGIZER

The energy needed to run our bodies actually comes from the energy of the sun that has been stored in food. Plants capture the sun's energy through a process called photosynthesis. This process combines sun energy with water and carbon dioxide to make carbohydrate, proteins and fats, also releasing oxygen to the air in the process. We, and other animals, breathe in the oxygen and eat plant food, and reverse this process. We convert food back into carbon dioxide, water and energy.

We need to metabolize energy from food for all of our life processes—everything from breathing to digestion to thinking to moving muscles. Metabolism is the process of life. It involves the breaking down of food carbohydrates, proteins and fats into smaller units, reorganizing these units as sources of energy, larger molecules and tissue building blocks, and eliminating waste products of the process. Lipoic acid is concerned with the catabolic portion of metabolism that breaks down the larger molecules (such as glycogen) into smaller molecules such as pyruvic acid. Specifically, lipoic acid is a key factor in converting food carbohydrates and fats into blood sugar (glucose) and fatty acids which then go through a process that leads to the extraction of energy. Lipoic acid is also involved in protein metabolism, but this is not a major energy pathway.

The body needs to "burn" blood sugar to produce energy, but instead of using high temperatures like those of a fire, the body has special biological catalysts called enzymes which extract the energy from sugars and fatty acids at normal body temperatures. Catalysts are atoms or molecules that facilitate reactions that either, as is the situation in the body, would not occur to any significant degree without their help, or in the case of commercial plant production, need to be sped up to be economically feasible. Catalysts are not consumed in these reactions, and a small amount can facilitate many cycles of the reaction that they facilitate.

Enzymes are proteins that act as catalysts and are not consumed in the process. They are there to facilitate the process along the way. As mentioned earlier, enzymes are made from coenzymes which in turn are often made from vitamins. Lipoic acid is a coenzyme that does not need a vitamin precursor.

Lipoic acid is a coenzyme for several enzymes. Lipoic acid is a coenzyme for both alpha-keto acid dehydrogenase complex enzymes (i.e., pyruvate dehydrogenase complex and alpha-ketoglutarate dehydrogenase complex), branched chain alpha-keto acid dehydrogenase complex, the glycine cleavage system, and Component X, which is associated with the pyruvate dehydrogenase complex, but its function is still unknown at this writing.

In essence, the body forms a multienzyme complex involving lipoic acid to break down molecules of pyruvate produced in earlier metabolism, into slightly smaller, high-energy molecules called acetyl-coenzyme A (acetyl-CoA). This results in molecules that can enter into a series of reactions called the citric acid cycle or Krebs cycle, which finishes the conversion of food into energy.

Sugars and fats are first harshly oxidized in the body by other enzymes that combine them with oxygen that we have breathed in through our lungs. These products must then be acted upon by the lipoic acid enzyme complex in order for the process to continue into the citric acid cycle.

Lipoic acid is involved in what is called a decarboxylation, which simply means that it cleaves off carbon dioxide. In the process excess energy is liberated which the body captures as ATP (adenosine triphosphate) and then uses that to provide the energy for muscle contraction.

Lipoic acid is a cofactor in a multienzyme complex that catalyzes what biochemists like to call "oxidative decarboxylation of alpha-keto acids," such as pyruvic acid. Forget the jargon and just remember that pyruvic acid is a product of a process called glycolysis, which is the first step in converting blood sugar (glucose) into energy that the body can burn. The lipoic acid itself, a coenzyme, is bound to a very complex enzyme which is a high molecular weight protein and as such it is not consumed when it is serving as a metabolic cofactor but it is continually regenerated.

The metabolic function of lipoic acid occurs inside cells. The processes that it catalyzes actually occur in the round and rod-shaped structures called mitochondria in the cytosol (interior) of cells. Mitochondria are sometimes called the "powerhouse" of the cell, where food is converted into energy.

In 1984, a Dr. Reuben reported a clinical condition resulting from abnormal lipoic acid coenzyme function. This condition gives us a "tool" for determining what would happen in a lipoic acid deficiency. Dr. Reuben described the hypotonia (reduced solute concentration), failure to thrive, reduced muscle mass, cerebral cortical atrophy and severe lactic acid accumulation caused by this disorder. Lipoic acid supplementation relieved these problems.

In 1990, Dr. L. Yoshida and colleagues at the University of California at San Diego reported that lipoic acid supplementation benefited a patient with defective enzymes of the multienzyme complex.

The reason for going through all this biochemistry is to make sure three "take-home" messages are clear. First, a shortage of lipoic acid would be a critical bottleneck slowing down the energy process. If a person lacks energy because of a deficiency in lipoic acid, supplemental lipoic acid will restore that person's energy level to normal. However, lipoic acid is not a stimulant like caffeine.

BLOOD SUGAR CONTROL

The second "take-home" message is that since lipoic acid facilitates the conversion of blood sugar into energy, it can have an effect on blood sugar level. Normally it is not the controlling factor for blood sugar level, because this entire process is subject to other types of enzymatic control. However, there is strong evidence that high intake of lipoic acid does influence glucose level. The high intake means a level that the body normally doesn't produce. This would be an effect of either diet or supplementation. It takes a consumption of more than 100 milligrams (preferably 500 to 600 milligrams) per day before any effect would be seen on glucose metabolism. Later on I discuss the research and experience gained through two decades of therapeutic use in Germany in the reduction of side effects in diabetes.

GLYCATION

The third message is that lipoic acid supplements which normalize blood sugar levels also reduce glycation. Glycation is the process in which proteins react with excess glucose. This sugar damage is just as detrimental to protein as is oxygen damage.

There is strong evidence that lipoic acid does keep the glucose level in the blood under control, and reduced levels of glucose mean less glycation. That is important in slowing aging and reducing diabetic side effects. The role of glycation in aging will be discussed in the section on aging.

PHYSIQUE ENHANCEMENT

For many of those with impaired energy production due to lipoic acid shortage, age or disease, supplementation may help restore the energy level to normal. Studies involving diabetics have shown that lipoic acid increases the amount of blood sugar converted into energy while not increasing the amount of blood sugar converted into fat. When people have their energy level restored, then they can exercise harder and longer. With increased exercise, there is increased muscle growth and more mitochondria to burn food calories and build muscle. Increased muscle size increases the basic metabolic rate, which in turn decreases body fat. Lipoic acid can thus have a favorable effect on body structure by promoting increased muscle size and decreased body fat.

SUMMARY

The three important messages in this section are:

1. Lipoic acid deficiency can be a bottleneck slowing energy production.
2. Lipoic acid supplementation can help normalize blood sugar
   . levels. This is extremely important to diabetics.
3. Lipoic acid supplementation reduces glycation, which damages proteins and accelerates aging.

PROTECTION AGAINST DISEASE

Lipoic acid's role as an outstanding, universal antioxidant is exciting many researchers today. The interest is so great because antioxidants help protect us from approximately 80 different age-related diseases. These diseases are not really caused by the mere passage of time, but by the cumulative damage done by free radicals to cell membranes and DNA.

It is becoming difficult to keep track of all of the diseases that are now linked to free radicals. Free radicals are highly reactive entities that occur in the body and do damage that leads to disease. The list of free-radical related diseases reads like the table of contents of a general medical text. A 1993 study by Pracon, Inc., of Reston, Virginia., concluded that if Americans took optimal amounts of just the three best known antioxidant nutrients—beta-carotene, vitamin C and vitamin E—we would save $ 8.7 billion annually from reduced hospitalizations for heart disease and cancer alone.

These free radical diseases include cancer, heart attacks, strokes, rheumatoid arthritis, cataracts, and Alzheimer's disease—the major cause of admission to nursing homes. The list keeps growing. Before Dr. Denham Harman's "free radical theory of aging," disease was mostly attributed to germs and aging—and aging was an unknown process. Although Dr. Harman's theory of free radicals and aging was developed in 1956, it wasn't until years later that other researchers linked other diseases to free radicals (e.g., cancer by Passwater in 1972 and heart disease by Steinberg in 1981.) Now we have disease pathologies involving free radicals that can be studied—and prevented, with the help of antioxidant nutrients such as lipoic acid.

It took a long while for the concept that free radicals could cause disease to be accepted. But it was also a long time before Louis Pasteur's germ theory was widely approved. A free radical is just as deadly as a germ, but in a different way. Of course, neither one germ nor one free radical presents a grave danger by itself. When germs infect a person—which usually happens only when their immune system is not functioning optimally—the germs (microorganisms such as viruses or bacteria) multiply and take over host functions. Free radicals also multiply and create chain reactions, and they do damage over time that alters body function.

Just as the wonder drugs—the antibiotics such as penicillin—cure killer infectious diseases, the wonder antioxidant nutrients can prevent killer diseases and help alleviate the symptoms and side effects of inflammatory diseases such as arthritis and even diabetes.

Antioxidant nutrients protect us from so many diseases because so many diseases involve free radicals and reactive oxygen species. Free radicals are molecules or fragments of molecules that are unstable and highly reactive. They are produced as the result of a normal molecule losing or gaining an electron.

In stable molecules, electrons normally associate in pairs. However, body processes such as metabolism can short-circuit the customary biochemical pathway, resulting in oxygen compounds that have lost an electron. This leaves each of these oxygen atoms or oxygen-containing molecules with an extra unpaired or lone electron. This is an oxygen free radical. Since the laws of nature work to restore atoms and molecules to their normal states, this oxygen atom becomes very reactive and seeks to regain an electron by grabbing one from another atom or molecule.

Several different types of oxygen radicals and other reactive oxygen species can be formed during normal metabolism. The table below lists the main oxygen radicals and reactive species. The hydroxyl radical is the most damaging radical to body components.

There are tens of thousands of free radicals created in the body every second. Critical body components such as DNA, the genetic material that directs the manufacture of each of our cells, can be altered by free radicals. The DNA in each cell may be hit about 10,000 times a day, according to Dr. Bruce Ames.

When one free radical captures an electron from another molecule, this creates a new free radical, as the second molecule now has a lone, unpaired electron. Of course, this new free radical will seek to capture another electron and become normal again. As you can see, this process could be never-ending. A free radical grabs electrons from another molecule, which then becomes a free radical and grabs another electron from still another molecule, and on and on—a chain reaction. Some of the compounds are altered by this process and portions of DNA or cell membranes are damaged. As a result, they don't function properly and health is impaired.

Unfortunately, free radical chain reactions can take place in your body countless times a day. To make matter worse, there are other sources of free radicals besides those generated during oxygen metabolism. Cigarette smoke, pollutants, sunlight, radiation, and even emotional stress can create free radicals and cause free-radical chain reactions.

Fortunately, you have powerful defenses against these free radicals. If you nourish your body properly, you can make ample quantities of antioxidant enzymes that will terminate these free radical reactions. Your main antioxidant enzyme defenses are superoxide dismutase, catalase and glutathione peroxidase. These antioxidant enzymes require trace minerals including selenium, manganese, copper, zinc and iron.

Your body also relies directly on other nutrients that are them-

Common free radicals and other reactive oxygen species of biological importance

Name	Conventional Symbol	Terminated by Lipoic acid	Terminated by dihydrolipoic acid
Superoxide anion	$O_2^{\bullet-}$	No	In question, probably not
Hydroxyl radical	$HO^{\bullet}$	Yes	Probably
Alkoxyl radical	$RO^{\bullet}$	?	?
Peroxyl radical	$ROO^{\bullet}$	Possibly, but not certain	Possibly, but in doubt
Hypochlorous acid	HOCl	Yes	Yes
Singlet oxygen		Yes	Yes (2 of 3 studies)
Hydrogen peroxide	H_2O_2	No	No
Transition metals	Fe, Cu, Cd, Pb, Hg	Chelates	Chelates

selves antioxidants to terminate free-radical reactions. Antioxidant nutrients have the ability to surrender electrons to rampaging free radicals without adding to the chain reaction. Thus, antioxidants can terminate reactive free radicals and, in turn, the antioxidant does not become a damaging free radical but a very sedate, low-energy, long lasting free radical that does no further harm to the body. Such antioxidant nutrients include vitamin A, vitamin C, vitamin E, mixed carotenoids, bioflavonoids and lipoic acid.

Dr. Lester Packer has elucidated the mechanisms responsible for the synergism of the major antioxidant nutrients. It turns out that there are antioxidant cycles, in which one antioxidant can regenerate or recharge another that has been altered in a free radical reaction and can no longer function as antioxidant. Each antioxidant does not necessarily act on its own, but often antioxidants have interconnected actions, which determine the antioxidant potency of the body or parts of the body. In the case of the redox-based antioxidants like the thiols (including the glutathione and lipoic acid systems), the vitamin C system and the vitamin E antioxidant cycle, there is clearly a synergism that exists when all three components are interacting with one another.

When a compound is reduced, it gains an electron. When a compound is oxidized, it loses an electron. Reducing power refers to a compound's ability to donate an electron, that is, to reduce another compound. If a compound donates an electron easily, it has high reducing power. If it hangs on tightly to electrons, it has low reducing power.

Lipoic acid has a low redox potential, which means that its reduced form, dihydrolipoic acid, very readily donates electrons to other compounds. So, for example, it can reduce oxidized glutathione to reduced glutathione. It also directly reduces the vitamin E radical, formed when vitamin E quenches lipid peroxidation, back to vitamin E. And it will reduce the semidehydroascorbyl back to ascorbate (vitamin C). That, in turn, links it to vitamin E, because vitamin C can also reduce the vitamin E radical. So you can see that all these antioxidants are tightly interlinked, with lipoic acid playing a role in recycling many of the key antioxidants in the cell.

When we talk about oxidation and reduction, there are always two compounds involved, one which loses an electron and one which gains an electron. For example, when vitamin E terminates lipid peroxidation, that's an oxidation-reduction reaction. Vitamin E donates an electron to a peroxyl radical. The vitamin E is oxidized and the peroxyl radical is reduced. "Redox" is just sort of a shorthand way of saying "reduction and oxidation," and redox cycles are groups of linked redox reactions. To take the vitamin E example again, after the vitamin E loses an electron, it can be given an electron by another compound, for example, vitamin C. Now the vitamin C has become oxidized, and the vitamin E is reduced—it's been cycled back to its original form.

We discussed earlier how its structure determines lipoic acid's antioxidant capabilities, but let's summarize its actions briefly here.

Lipoic Acid—the Ideal Antioxidant

Although there is no one, single perfect antioxidant, lipoic acid is a candidate that approaches that ideal. The antioxidant nutrients are partners working together. Vitamin C, vitamin E and vitamin A are essential vitamins as well as antioxidants. However, they work better when there is more lipoic acid available than what is tied up in use as a coenzyme. Dr. Packer has described an ideal antioxidant as one that has the following biochemical properties:

1) quenches free radicals
2) is easily absorbed and is readily bioavailable
3) concentrates in tissues, cells, and extracellular fluid
4) is present in more than one domain such as aqueous fluids, membranes, cytosol or lipoproteins
5) interacts with other antioxidants
6) chelates free metal ions
7) has positive effects on gene expression

The lipoic acid—dihydrolipoic acid redox couple does all of the above very well.

Lipoic acid can partially replace some of the dietary need for vitamin C and vitamin E. In 1959, Drs. Rosenberg and Culik showed that lipoic acid prevented scurvy in vitamin C-deficient animals, and that it prevented symptoms of vitamin E deficiency in laboratory animals fed a vitamin E-deficient diet. They even predicted that lipoic acid might act as an antioxidant for vitamin C and vitamin E.

Lipoic acid terminates the hydroxyl and hypochlorous free radicals and tests are divided as to whether or not it quenches the peroxyl free radical. Its reduced form, dihydrolipoic acid, also terminates hydroxyl and hypochlorous free radicals, but in addition also terminates superoxide free radicals and definitely quenches peroxyl free radicals. In addition, lipoic acid also quenches the reactive oxygen species singlet oxygen and possibly hydrogen peroxide in some domains but not in others. Results are not yet clear as to whether or not dihydrolipoic acid quenches singlet oxygen.

LIPOIC ACID INCREASES GLUTATHIONE LEVELS

As part of its regeneration of its partner antioxidant, lipoic acid also increases cellular glutathione content. Glutathione is a major antioxidant within cells. We will discuss this action of lipoic acid further in the sections on cataract and AIDS.

SUMMARY

Free radicals are major factors in about 80 diseases, including heart disease, cancer, aging, diabetes, arthritis, cataracts, Alzheimer's disease and many others. Antioxidants destroy free radicals and thus prevent these diseases. Antioxidant nutrients also help alleviate the symptoms and side-effects of many of these diseases. Lipoic acid approximates the ideal antioxidant because it is both water- and fat-soluble, works inside and outside of cells, participates in redox cycling, recharges other important antioxidants and quenches several free radicals and reactive oxygen species.

EFFECT ON GENES AND HEALTH

The excitement soared when it was found that lipoic acid can play a major role in protecting the genes that determine our health. I have been researching antioxidant nutrients since 1959 and I haven't seen this much excitement among researchers since the early days when we learned that free radicals cause many diseases. Now a whole new level of knowledge has been uncovered that explains so much more about why antioxidants in general, and lipoic acid in particular, protect against disease.

Today, we often read that a gene has been found that either causes or increases our susceptibility to develop this or that disease. Therefore, we tend to think that a great deal of disease is genetic in origin. We may rationalize that, since our family is prone to colon cancer or heart disease or whatever, then that's that—if it's all genetic, then why even bother with nutrition and exercise? Well, consider that the gene that causes a particular disease just sits there causing no trouble until hit by a free radical or a certain nuclear factor. Also consider that this gene won't be activated to do its damage if certain antioxidants prevent the free radical or nuclear factor from reaching the gene.

If a particular nuclear factor is activated, it can activate or damage genes, and this in turn determines our health. The discovery of this relationship has only very recently come to light and scientists are very excited as they realize more than ever that antioxidants have great implications for our health.

This section is about the new knowledge that extends our understanding of the role of lipoic acid from just terminating free radicals, but also to protecting the genes from damage from certain nuclear factors. The future may prove that this is the most important part of this Good Health Guide, even though it is short.

We can understand the role of lipoic acid with the introduction of just two concepts, genes and a nuclear factor. Free lipoic acid—that is not tied up as part of the multienzyme complex for energy production—has the ability to protect the genetic material, DNA, in the cell nucleus. A gene is a "block" (segment) of DNA that operates as a unit within a chromosome to control a specific cell function by regulating the production of a specific protein. There are about 100,000 genes in each of the 46 chromosomes in the nucleus of cells. Genes are capable of reproducing themselves at each cell division, and they are capable of managing the formation of body proteins through processes called gene expression and regulation. Any factor that interferes with normal gene regulation can profoundly influence health and lifespan. Free radicals and other reactive oxygen species can influence gene expression and regulation.

Genes can be activated by a protein complex called Nuclear Factor kappa-B (NF-kappa-B). This activator can bind to DNA in genes and cause changes in the rate of gene activation. Old animals, including man, have more NF-kappa-B bound to their genes than do young animals. The most-studied effect of NF-kappa-B has been its effect on the immune system, but it is also known to lead to such things as defective skin cells and aged skin, and apparently can also be responsible for defective cells in all organs, with consequent impaired function of all body systems.

This gene activator, NF-kappa-B, is held in check by other protein sub-units called I-kappa-B proteins. When an I-kappa-B protein binds to NF-kappa-B, the complex cannot pass from the cell cytoplasm through the porous two-layered membrane of the nuclear envelope into the nucleus where the genes are located. The goal for health is not to allow excess NF-kappa-B to be released from the complex, and to permit the body to control its release by normal processes. However, free radicals, peroxides, and ultraviolet energy can induce the inactive complex to dissociate and allow the NF-kappa-B to penetrate into the nucleus and damage DNA.

Antioxidants, by virtue of the fact that they can inhibit free radicals and other reactive oxygen species, are able to inhibit activation of this transcription factor. Lipoic acid is of particular interest because it is where the action is—in the cell interior, the cytosol. An advantage of lipoic acid is that it is a relatively very small molecule and is readily transported through cellular membranes, including the nuclear membrane. It can therefore not only terminate free radicals in the bloodstream and on the cellular membrane, but protect NF kappa-B in the cytosol and even protect the DNA in the nucleus.

The interaction of the redox couples of lipoic acid/dihydrolipoic acid and glutathione/reduced glutathione on the regulation of NF-kappa-B, tumor necrosis factor and the growth-regulating gene c-fos are complex. Future research will explain more about them and how lipoic acid can help us maintain optimal health.

This section is intended to give you an introduction to the role of lipoic acid and gene expression. Gene expression will be discussed further in the sections on cancer and AIDS. Now that we have covered how lipoic acid protects us against disease by terminating free radicals and protecting our genes, we can look at its role in specific diseases.

There are many benefits to slowing the aging process besides looking younger longer. A more important benefit is that slowing the rate at which your body ages also delays the occurrence of the so-called age-related diseases. In fact, they can be postponed right out of your lifespan! This section is about how we can achieve the goal of living better longer.

Although the aging process appears very complex when viewed as a group of specific chemical reactions, we can simplify matters by concentrating primarily on the loss of information in the molecules responsible for reproducing the body's proteins. Free radicals and glycation are the responsible culprits. We have already discussed free radicals. Glycation is the modification of a protein by the action of a sugar molecule. Lipoic acid is doubly protective against aging because it protects against free radicals and glycation.

Aging can best be described as the process that reduces the number of healthy cells in the body. Although we have noted the increase of some enzymes in the body, and the decrease of others, the most striking factor in the aging process is the body's loss of reserves needed to respond to a challenge to its status quo (homeostasis).

What causes the body to lose its capacity to respond to a threat? The disappearance of cells from organs and tissues means that there is less of an organ or body system to produce what is needed to counter the threat. The body loses its ability to reproduce some of its cells, and, as cells are destroyed, they are not always replaced. One by one, the cells disappear until there isn't enough of the working tissue left to handle the challenge.

In addition to the loss of cells, there is a stiffening of tissues. By the mid-1960s it became apparent to me that free radicals could produce cross-linking (which I'll discuss shortly) as well as other damage. Later, I learned that blood sugar could react with body proteins to change their chemical and physical characteristics and cause aging in several ways, primarily by cross-linking and stiffening tissues and organs. Together, the loss of cells and the linking or stiffening of tissues age our bodies.

In 1970, my aging research was sufficiently advanced so that the antioxidant combinations were granted patents in several countries. My main contribution was the concept of the biological synergism of the antioxidant nutrients. The synergism approach made the antioxidant approach practical for humans. Dr. Denham Harman had developed the free-radical theory of aging, but he was working with single nutrients that had to be taken in very large—and impractical—amounts. My unified theory of aging was presented to the 23rd meeting of the Gerontological Society in Toronto on October 21, 1970, and reported in *Chemical & Engineering News* on October 26, 1970.

One major process that accelerates aging occurs when oxygen radicals cause a change in body proteins to produce oxygen-damaged proteins. To lessen damage from radicals, one merely needs to optimize antioxidant nutrient intake. This approach has proved to be very effective against secondary aging effects, and can lead to an additional 5 to 15 years of life and disease prevention, depending on when an individual starts the program.

HOW FREE RADICALS ACCELERATE AGING

The aging of the body through its loss of cells is caused largely by free radical reactions. There are five main ways in which free radicals age the body.

1. Lipid peroxidation, in which free radicals damage fatty compounds, causing them to essentially turn rancid and to release more free radicals in a chain reaction.
2. Cross-linking, in which free radicals cause proteins and/or DNA to fuse together. DNA is the core of the genetic material that replicates the body components, and altered DNA can't make what the body needs. Instead, useless debris is formed which clogs the body's mechanism and wastes nutrients and other needed factors.
3. Membrane damage, in which free radicals destroy the integrity of cell membranes. This interferes with the cell's ability to absorb nutrients and expel waste products. Both events kill cells.

4. Lysosomal damage, in which free radicals rupture lysosome membranes. Lysosomes are enzymes that can digest just about anything except the membranes that store them. When the membrane sac that stores them is ruptured, the lysosomes spill into the cell interior (cytosol) and destroy critical parts including the nuclei and mitochondria. The cells will then die without being able to reproduce.
5. Miscellaneous free radical reactions form residues called lipo-fuscin or age pigment. These residues accumulate with time and interfere with cell function and the life process.

All five of these processes destroy vital cells, and with each cell removed from our vital tissues we become one cell older.

GLYCATION

Blood sugar (glucose) and other sugars called reducing sugars, such as fructose and ribose, react spontaneously—without the need for enzymes—with collagen, a major protein found in skin, blood vessels and connective tissue, and other proteins to form cross-linked sugar-damaged proteins.

The rate of sugar modification of proteins is proportional to sugar concentration. As we discussed earlier, the process of form-ing these sugar-damaged proteins is called glycation. The actual sugar-damaged proteins and complex derivatives of glucose them-selves are called advanced glycosylation end products, AGEs for short. That's not a bad acronym as AGEs lead to a prematurely aged body. AGEs are yellowish-brown fluorescent structures. Gly-cation can be compared to the browning reaction in toast and sliced apples. The formation rate of AGEs increases as the blood sugar level increases and the length of time the level is raised increases.

The spontaneous reaction of sugar with tissue proteins such as collagen and myelin is responsible for accelerated tissue aging in diabetics, is believed responsible for kidney damage, and is also involved in the atherosclerosis process, which are both common complications of diabetes. Dr. Anthony Cerami observed that gly-cation reactions also play a role in the normal aging of tissue. This observation led to his glycation hypothesis of aging. Recent studies show that diabetics as well as aging animals do indeed have in-creased concentrations of AGEs in their collagen. Of related interest is the fact that average blood sugar levels tend to rise with increasing age, owing to the fact that the tissues become less sensitive to the actions of insulin as we age. This reduced sensitivity is not just a loss of reserve due to aging and the loss of tissue, but directly involves the interaction of insulin and the tissues themselves.

The roles of oxygen- and sugar-damaged protein definitely explain much of the secondary aging effects and some of the primary aging process. It appears likely that, other factors being equal, high or widely fluctuating blood sugar levels increase the cross-linking of collagen and other important proteins. Conversely, maintaining precise blood sugar control at the optimal level throughout life should result in tissues that are "young for their age."

Synergism of Antioxidants and Antiglycation

Evidence also suggests that the antioxidant and glycation approaches may be synergistic. Remember, it is not a matter of simply living longer. Both free radical reduction and glycation reduction reduce the incidence of the aging diseases—including heart disease, arthritis and cancer. They are complementary approaches that enhance each other's benefits. Synergy is also involved. As an example, the protection against free-radical damage is more efficient with both approaches than through the actions of either alone.

Studies by Dr. Hans Tritschler at the University of Heidelberg in Germany have shown that the nonenzymatic joining of sugar to protein to form AGEs causes a release of oxygen radicals after binding to receptors.

Some types of cellular damage caused by radicals can be repaired by enzymes. Some enzymes are made solely to repair damage to cells caused by radicals and by high levels of blood sugar.

Antioxidants reduce the damage that radicals do to cell components and to the enzymes that repair cells by reducing oxygen modification of proteins. However, without the additional action to prevent the formation of sugar-damaged enzymes, these enzymes will become inactive and unable to repair cell damage. Even though the repair enzymes are protected by antioxidant nutrients, the damage caused by high blood sugar levels quickly becomes significant.

Lipoic acid reduces the protein damage that high blood sugar levels cause. With lipoic acid's antiglycation action to prevent the damage from blood sugar, and its antioxidant action to protect against free radicals, the minor damage that does occur can be repaired by the still-functioning enzymes. The result is that the cell is protected and the body does not become damaged and thereby one cell older.

SUMMARY

Lipoic acid reduces glycation and free radical damage. This should prove in the future to have profound practical implications for health and longevity.

The stability of the living system becomes progressively impaired by chemical reactions, not the passage of time. If we can control the rate of these deleterious reactions, we can control the aging process.

SUGGESTED READING

1. Plans for a large-scale study of possible retardation of the human aging process. Passwater, Richard A. The Gerontologist 10(3):11,28 (1970)

2. Human Aging Research, Part II. Passwater, R. A. and Welker, P. A. American Laboratory 3 (5) 21–26 (1971) also International Laboratory 37–40 (July/August 1971).

3. The free-radical theory of aging. Harman, Denham. J. Gerontol. 11:298–300 (1956)

4. The longevity factor: Chromium Picolinate. Passwater, Richard A. Keats Publishing, Inc., New Canaan, Conn. (1993)

5. The new supernutrition. Passwater, Richard A. Pocket Books, New York (1991)

HEART DISEASE PREVENTION AND TREATMENT

Lipoic acid helps prevent heart disease and should be used in its treatment. Through its metabolic role, lipoic acid can lower cholesterol levels by 40 percent, according to laboratory animal studies. In addition, via its antioxidant role, lipoic acid protects against heart disease by its action in the cholesterol carriers called lipoproteins. Research since the 1980s has shown that it is not so important how much cholesterol is in the blood—although that is a factor—but whether or not the carrier of cholesterol has been damaged.

I have been researching heart disease and antioxidant nutrients since 1972. My emphasis has been on vitamin E. Lipoic acid is of interest because it is now known that it plays an important role in maintaining vitamin E in the active form needed to protect against heart disease.

In 1972, I published, "Dietary cholesterol: Is it related to serum cholesterol or heart disease?" in *American Laboratory*. This report established that blood cholesterol was not related to dietary cholesterol in the majority of people, and that dietary cholesterol was poorly related to heart disease. This was heresy in those days.

In 1974, *Prevention* magazine allowed me to conduct a survey of 18,000 of their readers. The study was primarily designed to determine if vitamin E supplementation benefited heart patients. An unexpected finding was that not only did vitamin E benefit actual heart patients, it greatly reduced the incidence of heart disease. The data indicated that length of time that vitamin E was consumed was a more important factor than how much vitamin E was taken. These findings were published in several issues of *Prevention* magazine during 1976, and again in my 1978 book *Supernutrition For Healthy Hearts*.

In May of 1993, two Harvard University School of Medicine studies were published back to back in the *New England Journal of Medicine* showing that vitamin E supplementation over 100 milligrams per day reduced the risk of heart disease by more than 40 percent. (NEJM 1993; 328: 1449–56). One, led by Dr. Meir Stampfer, was a study of female nurses, while the other, led by Dr. Eric Rimm, was a study of male health professionals.

PROTECTING THE CHOLESTEROL CARRIERS

There are several mechanisms that explain why vitamin E directly protects, and lipoic acid indirectly protects, against heart disease. One of these is the protection vitamin E affords the cholesterol carriers called lipoproteins. So let's take a minute or two and discuss lipoproteins. What are they, what do they do and why do we care?

There is no questioning that deposits can form in arteries and reduce the amount of blood that can travel through them and also set the stage for blood clots to form. A heart attack occurs when the heart doesn't get enough blood to provide fuel and oxygen. The formation of a blood clot is called thrombosis. When a clot forms in a narrowed coronary artery, it is called a coronary thrombosis. When the blood clot shuts off the blood supply, the tissue that the artery is supposed to feed will die. When a coronary thrombosis starves a section of the heart (myocardium), this section of tissue will die. The death of tissue is called infarction, so that a heart attack is called a myocardial infarction, sometimes an acute myocardial infarction.

There are thus two main points to address in preventing a heart attack. First, prevent the deposit from forming, and second, prevent the blood from clotting. Vitamin E can do both, and thus offers two-stage protection against heart attacks.

Now let's consider how these deposits form. They are invariably called cholesterol deposits because they contain cholesterol, which makes them visible as white areas.

The deposits depend more on the condition of the cholesterol carriers than on the amount of cholesterol being carried. Cholesterol is a fatty material, and it is not soluble in blood, which is primarily water. Almost everyone knows that oil (fat) is not soluble in water. This is why we use soap to dissolve oil and grime from our hands and clothes. One end of the soap molecules has an affinity for water, while the other end has an affinity for fat. Thus, soap can grab a fatty material and carry it away in water.

This would not work too well in the body. So the body has designed a better transport system for fats in the bloodstream. Proteins have regions that are water-compatible and other regions that are fat-compatible. Our bodies assemble a group of proteins into a hollow ball—actually a sphere-shaped particle. The proteins are aligned in such a way that all the water-friendly ends are on the outside perimeter of the particle, and all the fat-friendly ends are on the inside.

This particle, called a lipoprotein, can now carry fatty compounds in its center, where they will be shielded from the water that is the major component of the blood. The liver packages fatty compounds such as fatty acids, triglycerides and cholesterol into lipoproteins called low-density lipoprotein (LDL) to transport them to the cells where they will be used. Then the liver sends out another carrier, called high-density lipoprotein, to retrieve any excess fatty materials not used. Cells can build receptors that grab either LDL or HDL as needed. The system is apparently perfect, cholesterol transport is under strict control, both to and from the cells.

However, LDL can become damaged by oxidation or free radicals due to insufficient antioxidant levels. Such damaged LDL is called oxidized-LDL (Ox-LDL). Ox-LDL is taken up by scavenger receptors in artery cells. A long process is triggered, which need not be discussed here, but the essence is that when Ox-LDL enters artery cells, the immune system sends monocytes to attempt to rid the cells of the damaged LDL. Some of these monocytes are converted into macrophages. Both macrophages and monocytes are white blood cells. Their appearance in the cells is called foam cell formation because this is what the lipid-laden white cells look like—foam in the artery cells. When more Ox-LDL enters the artery cells than can be handled by the monocytes, the cells become damaged and deposits build up. This discussion, of course, is an oversimplification, but it serves to illustrate that the big culprit in heart disease is inadequate antioxidants, not too much cholesterol. The cholesterol in normal LDL and HDL is not a factor in forming the deposits. It is primarily the cholesterol in the Ox-LDL that forms the deposits.

LDL cholesterol is often called the bad cholesterol while HDL cholesterol is called the good cholesterol. However, LDL cholesterol is "bad" only when it has been oxidized. The cholesterol carried in LDL, HDL and Ox-LDL is cholesterol. Cholesterol is cholesterol is cholesterol! It is only the condition of the lipoprotein particle that is carrying it that makes the difference.

Now what does all of this have to do with lipoic acid? The lipoproteins carry the fat-soluble antioxidant nutrients as well as the fatty materials. The fat-soluble antioxidants are carried along with the fats to protect them from oxidation. If we are well-nourished, our LDL doesn't become damaged. Vitamin E is the primary protector of LDL. However, vitamin E could quickly be consumed by free radicals if it didn't have antioxidant partners to protect it or recycle it back to its undamaged form, tocopherol.

Here's where lipoic acid comes in. Lipoic acid is transported in LDL with vitamin E. As we discussed earlier, lipoic acid can directly and indirectly recharge vitamin E so that it can keep on protecting LDL. In addition, lipoic acid directly protects LDL itself. Thus, lipoic acid offers double-barreled protection of LDL.

LIPOIC ACID IN THE TREATMENT OF HEART DISEASE

Several researchers in the former USSR have shown that lipoic acid lowers cholesterol in animals, notably Dr. V. E. Anisimov in 1969 and Dr. S. A. Koziov in 1971. The research that I report here is by Dr. V. N. Ivanov of the Department of Biochemistry of the Medical Institute of Chita in the former USSR in 1974. Dr. Ivanov noted that since lipoic acid favorably influences the metabolism of carbohydrates, proteins and fats, which are disturbed in heart patients, lipoic acid might be of value in lowering blood cholesterol. In 1960, Dr. C. Dojama found that lipoic acid was an antiatherogenic agent as it activated the oxioreductive enzymes involved in fat breakdown.

Dr. Ivanov used rabbits for his studies, because they were used for most of the prior cholesterol studies done around the world. He found that lipoic acid reduced total blood cholesterol by 40 percent and cholesterol in aortic tissue by 45 percent. He also reported that lipoic acid reduced blood LDL levels by 42 percent and aortic LDL levels by 45 percent.

The net result of Dr. Ivanov's experiments was that lipoic acid improved the amount of oxygen actually getting to the heart. Lipoic acid enhanced oxygen uptake in the heart by 72 percent, by 148 percent in the aorta, and by 128 percent in the liver.

Dr. Ivanov concluded, "The results achieved justify a recommendation of lipoic acid for wide usage in the treatment of patients with atherosclerosis."

SUMMARY

Lipoic acid protects against heart disease both via its metabolic role and via its antioxidant role. The dual roles of lipoic acid, the metabolic antioxidant, once again offer complete modes of protection. The results of Dr. C. Ivanov justify using lipoic acid in the treatment of heart disease.

CANCER

Today, it is fairly common knowledge that antioxidant nutrients protect against some cancers. The evidence began with laboratory animal studies decades ago and has been supported by epidemiological (population) studies. At this writing several clinical intervention studies are under way. When all of the evidence is in, perhaps by the year 2010 or so, we will have fairly definitive proof. What we have today is an appreciable body of evidence that unquestionably demonstrates that those who eat diets rich in fruits and vegetables are at lower risk to develop cancer. We also have reasonable evidence from animal, mechanistic and epidemiological studies that the protective factors in fruits and vegetables are primarily antioxidant nutrients including vitamin C, vitamin E, carotenoids, bioflavonoids and other antioxidant nutrients. While we wait for the final results, it is prudent to make sure that we get optimal amounts of the various antioxidant nutrients, including lipoic acid, which spares and regenerates its other antioxidant partners.

In this section, we will discuss how antioxidant nutrients in general protect against cancer, and how lipoic acid also protects the nuclear factor that prevents oncogene activation.

When I examined the incidence of cancer in my laboratory animals in my aging experiments, I did confirm a drastically lower incidence rate. I then conducted a series of experiments to study the possibility that the synergistic antioxidants were protective against cancer. They were.

In 1972, I filed for international patent protection for various combinations of nutrients that protected against cancer. I published my first results in *American Laboratory* in 1973 and have been issued patents on antioxidant synergism in the prevention of cancer. I continued my research and published *Supernutrition: Megavitamin Therapy* in 1975 and *Cancer and Its Nutritional Therapies* in 1978. This was updated as *Cancer Prevention and Nutritional Therapies* in 1993.

Even in the 1978 edition, I cited hundreds of studies that showed that the deficiencies of certain antioxidant nutrients increased the occurrence of both spontaneous and induced cancers. Conversely, many studies showed a dose-dependent relationship to lowered incidence of many cancers. That is, the more of the antioxidant nutrients consumed the greater the reduction in cancer rates. This, too, was shown for spontaneous and induced cancers.

WHAT IS CANCER?

Cancer is actually a group of diseases. There are 100 different types of cancers. What they have in common is that each is a disease of the body's cells. Most cancers involve tumors. Healthy cells grow, divide and replace themselves in an orderly way. A mutation can make cells lose their ability to limit and direct their growth. They divide too rapidly and grow without order. Too much tissue is produced and tumors are formed. Tumors can be benign or malignant. Malignant tumors are cancers, and they can spread and invade other parts of the body.

HOW LIPOIC ACID PROTECTS AGAINST CANCER

Lipoic acid can help keep cells from going astray. Earlier, we discussed how lipoic acid protected a complex called Nuclear Factor kappa-B, and prevented it from activating oncogenes. Oncogenes are genes that cause cancer. Oncogenes normally play a role in the growth and proliferation of cells, but when they are altered in some way such as by the activated NF kappa-B or a carcinogen, they cause the cell to become malignant. Dietary lipoic acid can enter the cytosol of cells and protect NF kappa-B from activation by radiation, free radicals or even sunlight.

We discussed earlier how antioxidants terminate free radicals. Free radicals can damage the sensors on cell membranes that signal the cell when to divide for growth. If the sensors are damaged, then unregulated growth can occur. Unregulated cell growth is the operative word in cancer.

If a free radical reacts with DNA in the nucleus, then the gene may produce an incorrect protein and the cell becomes altered or mutated. Free radicals can also impair the immune system, which would otherwise recognize and destroy mutated cells before they multiply and become cancer.

Since lipoic acid is a small molecule that is both water-soluble and fat-soluble, it can enter all body domains and terminate free radicals before they have a chance to cause the damage that can lead to cancer.

SUMMARY

Lipoic acid protects against cancer by protecting NF kappa-B from being activated to genes, and by its nearly universal presence as a powerful antioxidant to prevent membrane and DNA damage.

SUGGESTED READING

1. Cancer Prevention and Nutritional Therapies. Passwater, Richard A. Keats Publishing, Inc., New Canaan, Conn. (1993)

2. Molecular Medicine: Oncogenes. Krontiris, T. G. New Engl. J. Med 333(5) 303–6 (Aug. 3, 1995)

3. The genetic basis of cancer. Cavenee, W. K. and White, R. L. Sci. Amer. 72–9 (March 1995)

DIABETES

Lipoic acid is a very important nutrient for diabetics—it would not be an exaggeration to call it a blessing. Lipoic acid not only normalizes blood sugar levels in diabetics, it protects against the damage responsible for diabetes in the first place. It has been successfully used in Germany for more than 30 years, where it has reduced the secondary effects of diabetes, including damage to the retina, cataract formation, nerve and heart damage, as well as increasing energy levels.

Diabetes strikes one of every 20 Americans. Not only is it the third leading cause of death in the U.S., it inflicts serious suffering in the form of blindness, nerve damage, heart disease, gangrene, and amputated limbs. In little more than a generation, the incidence of diabetes has increased over 600 percent, accounting for 300,000 to 350,000 deaths each year during the early 1990s. About half of those with coronary artery disease and three-fourths of those suffering strokes developed their circulatory problems prematurely as a result of diabetes.

Diabetes is a group of diseases in which the body cannot properly metabolize food into energy. The result is a build-up of blood sugar that causes the long-term glycation damage we discussed earlier, and is responsible for even more immediate problems. The high sugar level in the blood results in osmotic changes and reduced blood volume, shock acidosis, coma and death. Insulin-dependent diabetes mellitus (type I) normally results when the body does not produce enough insulin. This is normally the result of damage to the beta cells of the pancreas. This form of diabetes usually, but not always, begins in childhood and was often called juvenile diabetes.

Non-insulin dependent diabetes (type II) accounts for about 85 percent of diabetes cases and is usually associated with age and/or obesity. It is still sometimes called adult-onset diabetes. This form of diabetes is caused by insulin resistance of peripheral cells or the inability of insulin receptors to utilize insulin efficiently. Usually, diet and oral medication can keep blood sugar levels near normal, but insulin is generally of no value. Type II diabetics generally have high levels of insulin in the blood, but it is ineffective because of the insulin resistance of the tissues.

Unhappily, even when blood sugar levels are reduced below a critical level, they still fluctuate widely and are still above the level that leads to glycation. Glycation damage and free radical damage lead to such diabetic complications as cataract, retinopathy, stiffened arteries and heart tissue, damaged lipoproteins (Ox-LDL) and nerve destruction.

Lipoic acid can terminate free radicals and thus reduce the oxidative stress that can damage the pancreas, cause cataracts, nerve damage, retinopathy and other side effects. Lipoic acid also reduces glycation, which otherwise can damage proteins, especially those of skin and blood vessels. Even more important to diabetics is that lipoic acid, by virtue of its ability to normalize blood sugar level and the entire glycolysis pathway for conversion of sugar into energy, allows the nerves to recover. Pain is reduced and normal feeling is restored.

Lipoic acid acts to increase glucose transport by stimulating the glucose transporters (a type of protein) GLUT-1 and GLUT-4 to move from the cell interior to the membrane. This action is independent of insulin transport. It is believed that the sulfur atoms of lipoic acid are responsible for the translocation action. This restoration of normal blood sugar level in turn increases the number of glucose transporters in the membranes of muscle cells. This is a very desirable cycle.

Lipoic acid supplementation at the level of 300 to 600 milligrams per day has been efficient in significantly lowering blood sugar, sorbitol, serum pyruvate and acetoacetate levels while increasing glycogen (stored energy compound for muscles) in muscles and the liver. At the same time, there is an increase in blood sugar utilization by muscle tissues and a reduction in liver glucose output.

IMPROVED NEUROLOGICAL FUNCTION

German studies with high doses of lipoic acid in diabetics have shown that it improves peroneal (leg) nerve conduction velocity, as well as heart and gastrointestinal functions. (See Reschke et al., item 13 in the reading list.)

Dr. D. Ziegler and colleagues at the Heinrich-Heine University in Dusseldorf, Germany have shown that long-term treatment with lipoic acid induces what is known as "sprouting," i.e., the growth of new nerve fibers in a regeneration process. In as little as three weeks there is a significant reduction in pain and numbness. The researchers observed no adverse effects from the high dosage (600 milligrams per day) of lipoic acid.

A review of the literature shows that in cell cultures, lipoic acid causes a dose-dependent sprouting of neurites in nerve cells. This has been attributed to improvement in nerve cell membrane fluidity. In animal experiments, lipoic acid promoted regeneration after partial denervation. Lipoic acid improves the blood flow in nerve tissues, improves glucose utilization in the brain and improves basal ganglia function.

In March, 1995, at an international meeting on diabetic neuropathy, in Munich, Germany, several researchers reported the results of clinical studies in which lipoic acid reversed the damage of diabetes to the nerves, heart and eyes of diabetics.

Most of the clinical studies were from European universities and clinics. Study after study reported that lipoic acid safely regenerated damaged nerves. The consensus was that lipoic acid protects through its antioxidant and antiglycemic actions. The conference concluded that lipoic acid was the agent of choice for the prevention of diabetic complications, including neuropathy, cardiomyopathy and retinopathy.

INCREASED MUSCLE ENERGY, DECREASED FAT PRODUCTION

At the Munich meeting Dr. Hans Tritschler's group reported additional information on how lipoic acid increases glucose uptake by muscle cells and decreases glucose uptake by fat cells. Dr. M. Khamaisi's group at the University of Negev in Israel reported that the increased glucose transport actually leads to increased energy production. This was confirmed with another study by Dr. Tritschler's group, using phosphorus magnetic resonance spectroscopic studies to show increased metabolism and ATP production in muscle tissues, and improved muscle recovery, which permits more work or exercise to be done.

The result is more energy production in muscles and less fat stored in the body. This is of course of special importance to diabetics who don't wish to, or can't, improve their lifestyle by exercising—but it is also obviously of great interest to everyone else!

CAUTION

Diabetics may require insulin or oral antidiabetic dose reduction to prevent hypoglycemic states. Close monitoring of blood glucose level is required.

SUMMARY

There is absolutely no doubt that all diabetics should be supplementing their diets with lipoic acid! It can mean all the difference in the world. They should also consider supplementation with chromium picolinate. It is imperative that diabetics monitor their blood sugar levels closely and have appropriate adjustments made to their medication doses to prevent lowering their blood sugar levels too far.

SUGGESTED READING

1. Lipoic acid as a biological antioxidant. Packer, L.; Witt, E. H. and Tritschler, H. J. Free Rad. Biol. Med. 19(2)227–50 (1995)

2. Lipoic acid and diabetes. Natraj, C. V.; Gandhi, V. M. and Menon, K. K. G. J. Biosci. 6:37–46 (1984)

3. Lipoic acid and diabetes. II. Gandhi, V. M.; Wagh, S. S.; et al. J. Biosci. 9:117–27 (1985). Lipoic acid and diabetes. III. Wagh, S. S.; Gandhi, V. M.; et al. J. Biosci. 10:171–9 (1986)

4. Mode of action of lipoic acid in diabetes. Wagh, S. S.; Natraj, C. V. and Menon, K. K. G. J. Biosci. 11:59–74 (1987)

5. Effect of lipoic acid and insulitis in nonobese diabetic mice. Faust, A.; Burkart, V.; et al. Int. J. Immunopharmac 16:61–66 (1994)

6. Dihydrolipoic acid protects pancreatic islet cells. Burkart, V.; Koike, T.; et al. Agents and Actions 38:60–5 (1993)

7. Stimulation of glucose utilization by thioctic acid. Haugaard, N. and Haugaard, E. S. Biophys. Acta 222:583–6 (1970)

8. Effect of lipoic acid. Singh, H. P. P. and Bowman R. H. Biochem. Biophys. Res. Com. 41:555–61 (1970)

9. Effect of thiotic acid on glucose transport. Bashan, N.; Burdett, E.; et al. In: Gries, F. A. and Wessel, K., eds. The role of antioxidants in diabetes mellitus. PMI-Verlag-Gruppe;1993:221–9

10. Chronic thioctic acid treatment increases insulin-stimulated glucose transport activity. Henriksen, E. J.; Jacob, S.; Tritschler, H.; et al. Diabetes. Suppl. 1:122A abstract; (1994)

11. Efficiency of thioctic acid in the therapy of peripheral diabetic neuropathy. Sachse, G. and Willms, B. Horm. Metab. Res. Supp. Ser 9:105 (1980)

12. Glucose transporters of muscle cells in culture. Klip, A.; Volchuk, A.; Ramlal, T.; et al. In: Draznin, B. and LeRoith, D., eds. Molecular biology of diabetes. Humana Press, Totowa, N.J. (1994)

13. High-dose long-term treatment with thioctic acid in diabetic polyneuropathy. Reschke, B.; Zeuzem, S.; Rosak, C.; et al. In: Borbe/Ulrich, eds., Thioctsaure: 318–34 (1989)

ADDITIONAL PROTECTION

Lipoic acid is important for many more reasons than can be included in this Good Health Guide. However, the role of lipoic acid in detoxification, cataract prevention, nerve regeneration, and the immune system enhancement that may prevent HIV infection from developing into clinical AIDS must be mentioned

DETOXIFICATION

It is apparent that lipoic acid is itself a versatile and direct antioxidant. However, there is still more to its antioxidant protective actions. It also has an indirect action via its ability to chelate many metals (minerals). To chelate means that a compound can grab a metal atom with "claws" formed by certain groups of atoms in the compound.

Iron and copper are essential nutrients, but excesses or "free" unbound atoms or ions can be harmful. If iron and copper are present in excess as free, unbound ions, they can be oxidants. Any compound that would chelate free ions of iron and copper would thus indirectly reduce oxidation and be considered an antioxidant. Lipoic acid does not chelate the desirable form of iron that is part of proteins such as hemoglobin or the enzyme catalase, but it appears to be capable of removing iron from the storage protein ferritin in both the ferrous and ferric states. I have not seen studies that would indicate whether lipoic acid would be of value to people with iron overload disorders, but there does seem to be some potential.

In most cases, iron and copper are complexed in the body with other proteins, so the concentration of free metal ions is quite low, but under some conditions of trauma, these metal ions can be released. When that happens, the ability to complex is very important, because that inhibits these ions' catalyzing oxidative processes.

Cadmium, lead and mercury are toxic metals at essentially all levels. Cadmium is a toxic metal that is present in tobacco smoke and accumulates in smokers. It is believed to be responsible for a significant amount of the harm caused by smoking. Lead is a toxic metal that gets into the air we breathe from automobile exhaust. It is also present in many water supplies and processed foods. Mercury is a toxic material present in dental fillings and in fish from mercury-polluted waters.

CATARACT

As we age, we are all at risk to develop cataracts, a degeneration of the eye lens. Diabetics are especially at risk, as they have increased oxidative and glycation damage. Excess exposure to sunlight is also a risk factor in the development of cataracts. The ultraviolet energy of sunlight creates free radicals in the tissues it impinges upon. The eye lens is directly exposed to sunlight, and, unfortunately, cells in eye lenses are not directly bathed by antioxidant-rich blood.

It is therefore difficult to keep these lens cells optimally nourished with antioxidant nutrients. Epidemiological studies have confirmed that persons with higher dietary intakes of antioxidant nutrients have a lower incidence of cataracts.

Lipoic acid is not only a powerful antioxidant that can get into cells easily due to its small molecular size and water and fat compatibility, it also facilitates glutathione production in cells. Glutathione is a major cellular antioxidant. Cataract tissues have low glutathione levels. In laboratory animal experiments, Dr. Lester Packer's group has shown that lipoic acid increased levels of glutathione, vitamin C and vitamin E in eye lens tissue (Free Rad. Biol. Med. 1994). Also, cell culture studies have shown that lipoic acid blocks cataract formation in lenses from diabetic rats.

AIDS

During HIV infection, key cells of the immune system called CD lymphocytes lose their ability to make and to transport glutathione. Since glutathione is a major cellular antioxidant, these immune cells succumb to oxidative stress and the immune system fails. As the immune system becomes impaired, the HIV-positive person increasingly develops opportunistic infections that ordinarily do not infect healthy people, and enters further into clinical AIDS.

This decline may·be prevented if the immune cells can keep their antioxidant status sufficiently high. Since lipoic acid is a powerful antioxidant and a facilitator of glutathione production, researchers conducted a small clinical trial that produced such exciting results, other larger studies are being planned at this writing.

Dr. J. Fuchs and colleagues gave 150 milligrams of lipoic acid three times daily for a two-week period and found that plasma glutathione levels increased in all patients, the number of T-helper cells increased in two-thirds of the patients, and the T-helper/T-suppressor cell ratio improved in 60 percent of the patients (Arzneimittel-Forschung 43:1359–62;1993).

A cell culture study found that lipoic acid prevented the replication of the HIV virus. The HIV virus replicates when NF-kappa-B is activated. We discussed earlier how lipoic acid protects NF-kappa-B from being activated which in turn causes genes to be expressed (to produce more of what it is supposed to produce).

NEURODEGENERATIVE DISEASES: NERVE REGENERATION, PARKINSON'S DISEASE AND ALZHEIMER'S DISEASE

In the section on diabetes, I discussed how lipoic acid improves nerve transmission and even regenerates nerves in diabetics. The effect of high blood sugar levels is to destroy nerves. The role of lipoic acid is more than just to allow the nerves to regenerate because it lowers blood sugar to normal in diabetics. It also improves membrane fluidity in nondiabetics. We have glycation aging us even if we don't have diabetes. Sugar-damaged proteins are just as harmful as oxygen-damaged proteins. Lipoic acid is protective against both glycation and oxidation. There is even more to the story to learn.

The central nervous system is especially vulnerable to oxidative damage because of its high oxygen consumption. The increased oxygen radical production increases mitochondrial dysfunction, which in turn increases radical production. This leads to cell death in brain and CNS tissue. In neurodegenerative diseases such as Parkinson's disease and Alzheimer's disease. mitochondrial dysfunction and oxidative stress may cause or worsen the clinical features. (Tritschler, H. J.; Packer, L. and Medori, R., Biochem. Mol. Biol. Int. 34:169–81;1994)

Lipoic acid is especially suited to protect nerve tissues against oxidative damage, and has been found to be neuroprotective. (Greenamyre, J. T.; et al., Neurosci. Letters 171:17–20;1994)

In animal studies, 100 milligrams of lipoic acid per kilogram of body weight improved memory even to the point better than that of young animals not given extra lipoic acid. (Stoll, S.; et al., Pharmacol. Biochem. Behav. 46:799–85;1993)

SAFETY

The miracles of lipoic acid would be of little value unless its use were safe. It is not a matter of more benefit than risk; it is a matter of *Primum non nocere:* First, do no harm.

Lipoic acid is made in the body and it is present in the diet. Food tables do not yet include the lipoic acid content of foods. Since lipoic acid is used in mitochondria, foods that are rich in mitochondria are good sources of lipoic acid. The most common foods rich in mitochondria would be red meats because they are some of the richest mitochondria sources. However, today people are deemphasizing red meat in their diets. Another good source of lipoic acid is yeast, which is not a staple of a typical American diet. Fortunately, lipoic acid supplements are available that are not derived from meat or animal products.

No clinical, toxicological or postmarketing studies have shown a serious adverse effect from lipoic acid supplementation, and it has been used for more than three decades at high dosage (300 to 600 milligrams per day) to treat diabetic neuropathy. However, as mentioned in the section on diabetes, diabetics will have improved glucose utilization and should monitor their blood sugar level closely and/or use it with the guidance of their physician.

Studies have not indicated any carcinogenic (cancer-causing) or teratogenic (birth defect) effects. However, as a precaution, until further information is available, lipoic acid supplements are not recommended for pregnant women.

Alcoholics or others who are severely deficient in thiamine (vitamin B1) should be sure to take thiamine supplements along with lipoic acid supplements.

As always with any food, there may be a few individuals who will have allergic-type responses such as skin reactions or upset stomach.

The acute toxic dose, expressed as LD50, is 400-500 milligrams per kilogram of body weight in several species. This is equivalent to 30,000 to 37,500 milligrams (30 to 37.5 grams) for a 165-pound human.

The typical prophylactic daily supplementation range for healthy adults appears to be 20 to 50 milligrams. Higher amounts may be recommended by health care providers according to the individual needs of their patients.